DR. BARBARA MUCUS CLEANSE

Revitalize your health: Dr. Barbara's proven mucus cleanse-discover effective methods to clear your system boost immunity and reclaim vitality

Miguel Sofia

Table of **Contents**

COPYRIGHT © 2023

CHAPTER ONE

Introduction to Dr. Barbara's Healing Method: Understanding the Importance of Mucus Cleansing in Health

In recent years, there has been a resurgence of interest in holistic approaches to health and wellness. Among these, Dr. Barbara's Healing Method has gained attention for its focus on mucus cleansing as a cornerstone of health. This method emphasizes the importance of addressing the accumulation of mucus in the body as a key factor in various health conditions and advocates for natural ways to cleanse the body of excess mucus.

Understanding Mucus and its Role in the Body

Before delving into Dr. Barbara's Healing Method, it's essential to understand the role of mucus in the body. Mucus is a viscous fluid produced by mucous membranes in various parts of the body, including the respiratory, digestive, and reproductive systems. Its primary function is to lubricate and protect these membranes from damage caused by irritants such as dust, bacteria, and viruses.

In the respiratory system, mucus helps trap foreign particles and pathogens, preventing them from reaching the lungs. In the digestive system, it lubricates food as it passes through the digestive tract and protects the stomach lining from digestive acids. Additionally, mucus in the reproductive system aids in the transport of sperm and provides lubrication during sexual intercourse.

While mucus plays a crucial role in maintaining the health of these systems, problems can arise when there is an excess buildup of mucus. This can occur due to various factors, including poor dietary choices, environmental toxins, and chronic health conditions. When mucus becomes thick and stagnant, it can impair the function of the organs and tissues it is meant to protect, leading to a range of health issues.

The Impact of Excess Mucus on Health

Excess mucus in the body can contribute to a wide array of health problems, ranging from mild discomfort to serious chronic conditions. In the respiratory system, it can lead to symptoms such as congestion, coughing, and difficulty breathing. Chronic respiratory conditions like asthma, bronchitis, and sinusitis are often associated with an overproduction of mucus and inflammation of the mucous membranes.

In the digestive system, excess mucus can interfere with proper digestion and nutrient absorption, leading to symptoms such as bloating, gas, and constipation. It can also contribute to the development of conditions like irritable bowel syndrome (IBS) and inflammatory bowel disease (IBD), where inflammation and mucus production are key factors.

Furthermore, excess mucus can affect other systems in the body, including the immune and lymphatic systems. When the body is burdened with toxins and waste products due to a buildup of mucus, the immune system may become overtaxed, increasing the risk of infections and autoimmune diseases. Similarly, impaired lymphatic drainage due to thickened mucus can hinder the body's ability to remove waste and toxins, leading to systemic inflammation and chronic health issues.

Dr. Barbara's Healing Method: An Overview

Dr. Barbara's Healing Method is a holistic approach to health and wellness that focuses on mucus cleansing as a central tenet. Developed by Dr. Barbara, a renowned naturopathic doctor and wellness expert, this method combines dietary modifications, herbal remedies, and lifestyle practices to support the body's natural detoxification processes and promote optimal health.

At the core of Dr. Barbara's Healing Method is the belief that many health problems can be traced back to an accumulation of mucus in the body. By addressing this underlying issue and supporting the body's innate ability to cleanse and heal itself, individuals can experience significant improvements in their health and well-being.

Principles of Mucus Cleansing in Dr. Barbara's Healing Method

Central to Dr. Barbara's Healing Method is the concept of mucus-forming and mucus-clearing foods. According to Dr. Barbara, certain foods have a tendency to increase mucus production in the body, while others have the opposite effect of promoting mucus clearance. By understanding the properties of these foods and making informed dietary choices, individuals can help reduce mucus buildup and support the body's detoxification processes.

Mucus-forming foods include dairy products, refined sugars, processed foods, and animal proteins. These foods are believed to contribute to excess mucus production and inflammation in the body, exacerbating existing health issues and impairing overall wellness. In contrast, mucus-clearing foods are typically plant-based and include fruits, vegetables, whole grains, and legumes. These foods are rich in fiber, antioxidants, and other nutrients that support detoxification and promote a healthy internal environment.

In addition to dietary modifications, Dr. Barbara's Healing Method incorporates herbal remedies and natural therapies to further support mucus cleansing and detoxification. Herbal teas, tinctures, and supplements are often used to help clear excess mucus from the body and promote the elimination of toxins through the lungs, digestive tract, and skin. Other detoxification practices, such as saunas, dry brushing, and hydrotherapy, may also be recommended to enhance the body's natural detox processes and support overall health.

Benefits of Dr. Barbara's Healing Method

Advocates of Dr. Barbara's Healing Method tout a wide range of benefits, including improved respiratory function, enhanced digestion, increased energy levels, and a stronger immune system. By reducing mucus buildup and supporting the body's natural detoxification processes, individuals may experience relief from chronic health issues such as allergies, asthma, digestive disorders, and autoimmune conditions.

Furthermore, proponents of this method often report improvements in overall vitality, mental clarity, and emotional well-being. By adopting a mucus-clearing diet and incorporating detoxification practices into their daily routine, individuals can experience a profound transformation in their health and quality of life.

Conclusion

In conclusion, Dr. Barbara's Healing Method offers a comprehensive approach to health and wellness that emphasizes the importance of mucus cleansing in promoting optimal health. By addressing the underlying issue of excess mucus in the body and supporting the body's natural detoxification processes, individuals can experience significant improvements in their physical, mental, and emotional well-being. Whether seeking relief from chronic health conditions or simply striving to achieve greater vitality and vitality, Dr. Barbara's Healing Method offers a holistic framework for reclaiming and maintaining optimal health.

CHAPTER TWO

The Role of Mucus in Disease: Exploring How Excess Mucus Contributes to Illness and Discomfort

Mucus, though often overlooked, plays a pivotal role in maintaining the health and integrity of various bodily systems. It serves as a protective barrier against pathogens, irritants, and foreign particles, particularly in the respiratory and digestive systems. However, when produced in excess or not properly cleared from the body, mucus can contribute to the development and exacerbation of a wide range of diseases and discomforts. In this exploration, we will delve into the multifaceted ways in which excess mucus contributes to illness and discomfort, spanning respiratory ailments, gastrointestinal disorders, and systemic conditions.

Respiratory Ailments

Excessive mucus production and retention in the respiratory tract can lead to a plethora of respiratory ailments, ranging from the common cold to chronic conditions like asthma and chronic obstructive pulmonary disease (COPD). When the respiratory mucosa becomes irritated or inflamed, it triggers an increase in mucus secretion as a protective response. While this increase in mucus production initially serves to trap and eliminate pathogens, chronic exposure to irritants or infections can result in an overproduction of mucus that overwhelms the body's clearance mechanisms.

In conditions such as bronchitis and sinusitis, excessive mucus production can obstruct the airways, causing symptoms such as coughing, wheezing, congestion, and difficulty breathing. Moreover, the accumulation of mucus provides an ideal environment for bacterial or viral growth, further exacerbating respiratory infections and inflammation. Chronic inflammation of the respiratory mucosa, as seen in conditions like asthma, perpetuates a cycle of mucus hypersecretion and airway constriction, leading to persistent symptoms and decreased lung function.

Gastrointestinal Disorders

In the gastrointestinal tract, mucus serves as a protective barrier that lubricates and shields the mucosal lining from abrasive substances and digestive enzymes. However, disruptions in mucin production or alterations in the composition of mucus can contribute to the development of gastrointestinal disorders. Conditions such as gastroesophageal reflux disease (GERD), gastritis, and inflammatory bowel disease (IBD) are characterized by inflammation of the gastrointestinal mucosa and increased mucus production.

Excessive mucus secretion in the stomach can lead to symptoms such as heartburn, nausea, and abdominal discomfort, as it interferes with the normal functioning of the gastric mucosa. In the intestines, abnormal mucus production can contribute to the formation of mucus plugs, which obstruct the passage of stool and lead to constipation or bowel obstructions. Furthermore, alterations in the mucosal barrier function and mucus composition may increase susceptibility to bacterial infections and exacerbate intestinal inflammation in conditions like Crohn's disease and ulcerative colitis.

Systemic Conditions

Beyond its localized effects, excess mucus production can have systemic implications, contributing to the development and progression of various chronic diseases. Prolonged exposure to inflammatory mediators and oxidative stress, secondary to chronic mucus hypersecretion, can promote systemic inflammation and oxidative damage throughout the body. This systemic inflammation is implicated in the pathogenesis of numerous chronic diseases, including cardiovascular disease, metabolic syndrome, and neurodegenerative disorders.

Moreover, the accumulation of mucus in the body can impair the function of the immune system, compromising its ability to mount an effective defense against pathogens and foreign invaders. Chronic mucus hypersecretion may also disrupt the balance of the microbiota in mucosal surfaces, leading to dysbiosis and increased susceptibility to infections. In individuals with compromised immune function, such as those with HIV/AIDS or undergoing immunosuppressive therapy, excessive mucus production poses a heightened risk of opportunistic infections and disease progression.

Conclusion

In conclusion, excess mucus production and retention in the body can contribute to a myriad of diseases and discomforts, spanning respiratory ailments, gastrointestinal disorders, and systemic conditions. Whether as a result of chronic inflammation, mucosal irritation, or alterations in mucus composition, excessive mucus production disrupts normal physiological processes and undermines the body's ability to maintain health and homeostasis. Recognizing the role of mucus in disease pathogenesis underscores the importance of targeted therapeutic interventions aimed at restoring mucus homeostasis and alleviating symptoms associated with mucus-related disorders. By addressing the underlying mechanisms driving mucus hypersecretion and promoting mucus clearance, clinicians can help mitigate the burden of mucus-related diseases and improve the overall health and well-being of affected individuals.

CHAPTER THREE

Dr. Barbara's Approach to Healing: Embracing Herbal Remedies for Mucus Reduction and Detoxification

Dr. Barbara's holistic approach to healing emphasizes the importance of mucus reduction and detoxification for achieving optimal health and wellness. Central to her methodology are herbal remedies, which have long been used in traditional medicine systems worldwide for their therapeutic properties. Dr. Barbara advocates for the incorporation of specific herbs known for their mucus-reducing and detoxifying effects into one's daily regimen. In this exploration, we delve into Dr. Barbara's approach to healing through herbal remedies, highlighting their roles in mucus reduction and detoxification.

Understanding Herbal Medicine in Dr. Barbara's Healing Method

Herbal medicine, also known as botanical medicine or phytotherapy, involves the use of plants and plant extracts for medicinal purposes. Throughout history, herbs have been revered for their diverse pharmacological actions and therapeutic benefits. In Dr. Barbara's Healing Method, herbal remedies play a central role in supporting the body's natural detoxification processes and reducing excess mucus accumulation.

Dr. Barbara emphasizes the importance of selecting herbs that possess mucus-reducing, expectorant, and detoxifying properties. These herbs work synergistically to help clear congestion, support respiratory function, and promote the elimination of toxins from the body. By incorporating herbal remedies into one's daily routine, individuals can enhance their overall health and well-being while addressing underlying imbalances contributing to mucus-related symptoms.

Key Herbs for Mucus Reduction and Detoxification

Several herbs stand out in Dr. Barbara's Healing Method for their effectiveness in reducing mucus production, promoting expectoration, and supporting detoxification. Among these key herbs are:

1. **Licorice Root (Glycyrrhiza glabra):** Licorice root is prized for its demulcent and expectorant properties, making it useful for soothing irritated mucous membranes and promoting the expulsion of mucus from the respiratory tract. It also exhibits anti-inflammatory effects, which can help alleviate symptoms associated with respiratory conditions such as bronchitis and asthma.

2. **Eucalyptus (Eucalyptus globulus):** Eucalyptus is renowned for its decongestant and antiseptic properties, making it a popular choice for respiratory health. Inhalation of

eucalyptus essential oil can help clear nasal congestion, reduce phlegm production, and ease breathing. Additionally, eucalyptus leaf tea can be used as a soothing expectorant for respiratory discomfort.

3. **Ginger (Zingiber officinale):** Ginger is prized for its warming and stimulating properties, which can help alleviate congestion and promote circulation. It also possesses anti-inflammatory and antioxidant properties, making it beneficial for reducing inflammation and supporting detoxification processes in the body. Ginger tea is commonly used to relieve respiratory congestion and aid digestion.

4. **Turmeric (Curcuma longa):** Turmeric is revered for its potent anti-inflammatory and antioxidant properties, attributed to its active compound, curcumin. It helps reduce inflammation in the respiratory tract, improve lung function, and alleviate symptoms of respiratory conditions such as asthma and bronchitis. Additionally, turmeric supports liver detoxification pathways, aiding in the elimination of toxins from the body.

5. **Peppermint (Mentha piperita):** Peppermint is valued for its cooling and soothing properties, making it effective for relieving respiratory congestion and discomfort. Menthol, the primary active compound in peppermint, acts as a natural decongestant, helping to clear nasal passages and

alleviate sinus pressure. Peppermint tea or steam inhalation with peppermint oil can provide relief from respiratory symptoms.

Incorporating Herbal Remedies into Daily Routine

In Dr. Barbara's Healing Method, herbal remedies are incorporated into one's daily routine to support mucus reduction and detoxification. This may involve the preparation of herbal teas, tinctures, capsules, or topical preparations, depending on individual preferences and needs. Herbal remedies can be used preventatively to maintain optimal health or therapeutically to address specific health concerns.

To incorporate herbal remedies into your daily routine, consider the following suggestions:

1. **Herbal Teas:** Brew herbal teas using dried herbs or tea bags and enjoy them throughout the day. Choose herbal blends that promote mucus reduction and detoxification, such as licorice root, ginger, and peppermint.

2. **Tinctures:** Take herbal tinctures diluted in water or juice as directed by a healthcare practitioner. Tinctures provide a concentrated form of herbal extracts and are convenient for on-the-go use.

3. **Capsules or Tablets:** Take herbal supplements in capsule or tablet form for targeted support. Look for standardized herbal extracts or formulations specifically designed to support respiratory health and detoxification.

4. **Topical Preparations:** Use herbal preparations such as chest rubs or inhalation balms containing menthol, eucalyptus, and other respiratory-supportive herbs. Apply topically to the chest, back, or throat to help relieve respiratory congestion and discomfort.

5. **Herbal Steam Inhalation:** Add a few drops of essential oils or dried herbs to hot water and inhale the steam to clear nasal congestion and promote respiratory health. Herbs such as eucalyptus, peppermint, and thyme are particularly beneficial for steam inhalation.

Conclusion

In conclusion, Dr. Barbara's approach to healing embraces the use of herbal remedies for mucus reduction and detoxification. By harnessing the therapeutic properties of key herbs, individuals can support their body's natural detoxification processes, alleviate respiratory symptoms, and promote overall health and well-being. Whether enjoyed as herbal teas, tinctures, capsules, or topical preparations, herbal remedies offer a safe and effective means of enhancing health and vitality. Incorporating herbal remedies into one's daily routine empowers individuals to take charge of their health and embark on a journey toward holistic wellness.

CHAPTER FOUR

Understanding the Body's Elimination Pathways: How Mucus is Generated and Expelled

Mucus, often overlooked and underappreciated, plays a crucial role in the body's elimination pathways, serving as a protective barrier and aiding in the removal of waste, toxins, and pathogens. Understanding how mucus is generated and expelled is essential for maintaining optimal health and supporting the body's natural detoxification processes. In this exploration, we delve into the intricacies of mucus production and expulsion, shedding light on the body's remarkable ability to eliminate harmful substances and maintain homeostasis.

Mucus Production: Origins and Composition

Mucus is a gel-like substance produced by specialized cells known as goblet cells, which are found in mucous membranes throughout the body. These mucous membranes line various organs and cavities, including the respiratory tract, digestive tract, reproductive organs, and urinary tract. Mucus secretion is regulated by a complex interplay of signaling molecules, hormones, and neural inputs, ensuring its production is finely tuned to meet the body's needs.

The composition of mucus varies depending on its location and function within the body. In the respiratory tract, mucus acts as a sticky trap, capturing airborne particles, pathogens, and pollutants before they can reach the lungs. It is composed primarily of water, mucins (glycoproteins), electrolytes, and immune cells, forming a viscous gel that can be expelled through coughing or sneezing.

In the digestive tract, mucus serves as a lubricant and protective barrier, facilitating the passage of food through the gastrointestinal tract and shielding the mucosal lining from digestive enzymes and abrasive substances. It contains mucins, electrolytes, antimicrobial peptides, and antibodies, forming a gel layer that helps maintain gut integrity and supports nutrient absorption.

Mucus Expulsion: Mechanisms and Pathways

Once generated, mucus must be effectively expelled from the body to prevent its accumulation and maintain healthy mucosal function. The body employs several mechanisms and pathways for mucus expulsion, each tailored to the specific anatomical location and physiological requirements.

In the respiratory tract, mucus clearance is primarily achieved through the coordinated action of cilia, tiny hair-like structures that line the respiratory epithelium. Ciliary movement, known as mucociliary clearance, propels mucus upward towards the throat, where it can be swallowed or expectorated. Additionally, coughing and sneezing serve as protective reflexes to expel excess mucus and clear the airways of foreign particles and pathogens.

In the digestive tract, mucus expulsion occurs through peristalsis, the rhythmic contraction and relaxation of smooth muscle in the intestinal wall. Peristaltic waves move mucus along the gastrointestinal tract, facilitating its elimination with feces. Additionally, the secretion of digestive enzymes and bile helps break down mucus and facilitate its passage through the digestive system.

In both the respiratory and digestive systems, proper hydration plays a critical role in mucus expulsion. Adequate fluid intake helps maintain mucus viscosity and hydration, facilitating its movement and clearance from the body. Conversely, dehydration can lead to thickened, inspissated mucus that is difficult to expel, increasing the risk of congestion, obstruction, and inflammation.

Factors Affecting Mucus Production and Clearance

Several factors can influence mucus production and clearance, impacting the body's ability to eliminate waste and toxins effectively. Chronic inflammation, allergies, infections, and environmental exposures can stimulate goblet cell hyperplasia and increase mucus production in the respiratory and digestive tracts. Conversely, conditions such as dehydration, smoking, and certain medications can impair mucociliary clearance and hinder mucus expulsion.

Moreover, dietary factors play a significant role in mucus production and composition. Certain foods, such as dairy products, refined sugars, and processed foods, are believed to increase mucus secretion and promote inflammation in susceptible individuals. In contrast, a diet rich in fruits, vegetables, whole grains, and healthy fats can support mucosal health and promote mucus clearance through its antioxidant, anti-inflammatory, and fiber-rich constituents.

Conclusion

In conclusion, understanding the body's elimination pathways and the role of mucus in waste removal and detoxification is essential for maintaining optimal health and well-being. Mucus serves as a critical barrier and clearance mechanism, trapping pathogens, toxins, and waste products before they can cause harm to the body. Through coordinated mechanisms such as mucociliary clearance and peristalsis, the body expels mucus and its contents, ensuring the integrity of mucosal surfaces and supporting overall health.

Factors that influence mucus production and clearance, including inflammation, hydration status, and dietary factors, can impact the body's ability to eliminate waste effectively. By supporting mucosal health through lifestyle interventions such as hydration, dietary modifications, and avoidance of environmental toxins, individuals can optimize mucus production and clearance, promoting detoxification and maintaining homeostasis.

CHAPTER FIVE

The Ultimate Herbal Mucus Cleanse Protocol: Step-by-Step Guide to Implementing Dr. Barbara's Program

Embarking on a herbal mucus cleanse protocol inspired by Dr. Barbara's approach to health and wellness requires a systematic and comprehensive strategy. This step-by-step guide outlines the key components of Dr. Barbara's program, providing a roadmap for implementing an effective herbal mucus cleanse protocol.

Step 1: Preparation and Planning

Before diving into the herbal mucus cleanse protocol, it's essential to set clear goals and establish a plan of action. Begin by assessing your current health status, identifying any symptoms or conditions related to excess mucus production, and determining your desired outcomes for the cleanse. Consult with a qualified healthcare practitioner or herbalist to ensure the protocol is suitable for your individual needs and health status.

Next, gather the necessary supplies and ingredients for the cleanse, including herbal remedies, dietary supplements, and supportive tools such as a juicer, blender, and herbal teas. Create a detailed meal plan and shopping list that emphasizes whole, unprocessed foods and includes plenty of fruits, vegetables, whole grains, and legumes. Consider gradually transitioning to a mucus-clearing diet in the days leading up to the cleanse to minimize discomfort and support detoxification.

Step 2: Herbal Support for Mucus Reduction

Central to Dr. Barbara's herbal mucus cleanse protocol is the incorporation of specific herbs known for their mucus-reducing and detoxifying properties. Choose high-quality herbal remedies from reputable sources and follow dosage recommendations provided by healthcare practitioners or product labels. Consider incorporating the following herbs into your cleanse:

- Licorice Root: Supports respiratory health and soothes irritated mucous membranes.

- Eucalyptus: Acts as a decongestant and expectorant, helping to clear respiratory congestion.

- Ginger: Provides anti-inflammatory and digestive support, aiding in mucus reduction and detoxification.

- Turmeric: Offers potent antioxidant and anti-inflammatory properties, supporting liver detoxification and reducing systemic inflammation.

- Peppermint: Relieves respiratory congestion and soothes digestive discomfort, promoting mucus clearance and detoxification.

These herbs can be consumed in various forms, including herbal teas, tinctures, capsules, and topical preparations. Experiment with different formulations and delivery methods to find what works best for you and your preferences.

Step 3: Dietary Modifications

In conjunction with herbal support, dietary modifications play a crucial role in Dr. Barbara's mucus cleanse protocol. Focus on eliminating mucus-forming foods such as dairy products, refined sugars, processed foods, and animal proteins, which can contribute to excess mucus production and inflammation. Instead, emphasize mucus-clearing foods such as fruits, vegetables, whole grains, and legumes, which are rich in fiber, antioxidants, and essential nutrients.

Consider incorporating the following dietary practices into your cleanse:

- Increase your intake of hydrating fluids such as water, herbal teas, and freshly pressed juices to support mucus clearance and detoxification.

- Include plenty of leafy greens, cruciferous vegetables, and antioxidant-rich foods in your meals to promote liver detoxification and reduce inflammation.

- Experiment with mucus-clearing soups, broths, and smoothies containing ingredients like ginger, turmeric, garlic, and leafy greens to support respiratory and digestive health.

Step 4: Lifestyle Support

In addition to herbal and dietary interventions, lifestyle modifications can further enhance the effectiveness of Dr. Barbara's mucus cleanse protocol. Prioritize rest and relaxation, engage in stress-reducing activities such as meditation, yoga, and deep breathing exercises to support the body's natural detoxification processes. Incorporate regular physical activity into your routine to promote circulation, lymphatic drainage, and overall well-being.

Avoid exposure to environmental toxins, pollutants, and allergens that can exacerbate mucus-related symptoms and compromise detoxification pathways. Practice mindful breathing techniques and steam inhalation with essential oils such as eucalyptus, peppermint, and lavender to soothe respiratory discomfort and promote mucus clearance.

Step 5: Monitoring and Adjustments

Throughout the herbal mucus cleanse protocol, listen to your body and monitor your symptoms and progress closely. Keep a journal to track changes in energy levels, digestion, respiratory function, and overall well-being. Adjust your herbal regimen, dietary choices, and lifestyle practices as needed based on your individual response and feedback from healthcare practitioners.

Be patient and gentle with yourself during the cleanse, recognizing that detoxification is a gradual process that takes time. Celebrate small victories and milestones along the way, and acknowledge the positive changes occurring within your body and mind. After completing the cleanse, gradually reintroduce foods and habits while continuing to prioritize mucus-clearing foods and supportive practices for long-term health and vitality.

Conclusion

In conclusion, Dr. Barbara's ultimate herbal mucus cleanse protocol offers a comprehensive and systematic approach to reducing excess mucus production and supporting detoxification. By incorporating specific herbs, dietary modifications, lifestyle practices, and supportive tools, individuals can optimize their body's natural elimination pathways and promote overall health and well-being. With careful planning, preparation, and commitment, the herbal mucus cleanse protocol provides a transformative opportunity to reset, rejuvenate, and reclaim optimal health.

CHAPTER SIX

Identifying Mucus-Forming Foods: Learning Which Foods to Avoid for Optimal Cleansing

In the pursuit of optimal health and wellness, understanding the impact of dietary choices on mucus production is essential. Certain foods have been identified as mucus-forming, meaning they have the potential to increase mucus production and contribute to congestion, inflammation, and other mucus-related symptoms. By learning to identify and avoid mucus-forming foods, individuals can support their body's natural cleansing processes and promote overall well-being. In this exploration, we delve into the characteristics of mucus-forming foods and provide guidance on making informed dietary choices for optimal cleansing.

Understanding Mucus-Forming Foods

Mucus-forming foods are those that have the potential to stimulate mucus production or exacerbate existing mucus-related symptoms. These foods may contain compounds or allergens that irritate mucous membranes, trigger inflammatory responses, or disrupt mucosal integrity. While individual responses to mucus-forming foods can vary, certain dietary patterns and food groups are commonly associated with increased mucus production and respiratory or digestive discomfort.

Common Mucus-Forming Foods to Avoid

1. **Dairy Products:** Dairy products such as milk, cheese, yogurt, and ice cream are notorious for their mucus-forming properties. Dairy contains casein and whey proteins, which some individuals may be sensitive to or have difficulty digesting. Additionally, lactose, the sugar found in dairy, can ferment in the gut and contribute to bloating, gas, and mucus production.

2. **Refined Sugars and Sweets:** Refined sugars and sweets, including candy, pastries, sodas, and sugary desserts, can promote inflammation and mucus production in susceptible individuals. These foods provide little nutritional value and can disrupt blood sugar levels, leading to energy crashes and cravings for more sugar.

3. **Processed Foods:** Processed foods such as packaged snacks, fast food, and convenience meals often contain artificial additives, preservatives, and flavorings that can irritate mucous membranes and trigger inflammatory responses. These foods are typically high in sodium, refined carbohydrates, and unhealthy fats, contributing to mucus formation and systemic inflammation.

4. **Animal Proteins:** Animal proteins such as red meat, poultry, and seafood can be mucus-forming for some individuals, particularly when consumed in excessive amounts or in

processed forms such as deli meats and sausages. Animal proteins are often high in saturated fats and cholesterol, which can promote inflammation and mucus production in the body.

5. **Gluten-Containing Grains:** Gluten-containing grains such as wheat, barley, and rye contain proteins known as gluten, which can be difficult to digest for some individuals and may trigger inflammatory responses in the gut. Gluten sensitivity or intolerance can manifest as digestive discomfort, bloating, and increased mucus production in susceptible individuals.

6. **Highly Acidic Foods:** Highly acidic foods such as citrus fruits, tomatoes, and vinegar-based condiments can irritate mucous membranes and exacerbate acid reflux or digestive discomfort in some individuals. While these foods can be part of a healthy diet in moderation, excessive consumption may contribute to mucus formation and digestive issues.

Making Informed Dietary Choices for Optimal Cleansing

To support optimal cleansing and reduce mucus-related symptoms, consider incorporating the following dietary practices:

- **Emphasize Whole, Plant-Based Foods:** Focus on whole, unprocessed plant foods such as fruits, vegetables, whole grains, legumes, nuts, and seeds. These foods are rich in fiber, antioxidants, vitamins, and minerals, supporting digestive health, reducing inflammation, and promoting mucus clearance.

- **Hydrate with Water and Herbal Teas:** Stay hydrated by drinking plenty of water throughout the day and enjoy herbal teas such as ginger, peppermint, and licorice root, which have mucus-clearing and soothing properties.

- **Limit Mucus-Forming Foods:** Reduce or eliminate mucus-forming foods from your diet, especially if you experience mucus-related symptoms such as congestion, coughing, or digestive discomfort. Experiment with an elimination diet to identify trigger foods and sensitivities, and gradually reintroduce foods while monitoring your body's response.

- **Choose Healthy Fats:** Include sources of healthy fats such as avocados, olive oil, nuts, and seeds in your diet to support mucosal integrity, reduce inflammation, and promote detoxification.

- **Support Digestive Health:** Incorporate fermented foods such as sauerkraut, kimchi, and yogurt with live cultures to support gut health and digestion. Consider taking probiotic supplements to replenish beneficial gut bacteria and improve digestive function.

- **Listen to Your Body:** Pay attention to how your body responds to different foods and dietary patterns, and adjust your diet accordingly. Practice mindful eating, chewing food thoroughly, and eating in a relaxed environment to support optimal digestion and nutrient absorption.

Conclusion

In conclusion, identifying and avoiding mucus-forming foods is an important aspect of promoting optimal cleansing and supporting overall health and wellness. By prioritizing whole, plant-based foods, staying hydrated, and limiting mucus-forming foods, individuals can reduce mucus production, alleviate mucus-related symptoms, and support the body's natural detoxification processes. Making informed dietary choices and listening to your body's cues are key steps in optimizing health and achieving balance in the body's elimination pathways.

CHAPTER SEVEN

Herbal Selection and Preparation: Identifying Key Ingredients for Mucus-Fighting Remedies

In the pursuit of mucus reduction and optimal health, herbal remedies play a pivotal role in supporting the body's natural detoxification processes. By selecting and preparing specific herbs known for their mucus-fighting properties, individuals can harness the therapeutic benefits of nature to alleviate congestion, promote respiratory health, and support overall well-being. In this guide, we explore the key ingredients for mucus-fighting remedies and provide guidance on their selection and preparation.

Identifying Key Ingredients for Mucus-Fighting Remedies

1. **Licorice Root (Glycyrrhiza glabra):** Licorice root is prized for its demulcent and expectorant properties, making it a valuable ingredient in mucus-fighting remedies. It helps soothe irritated mucous membranes, reduce inflammation, and promote the expulsion of mucus from the respiratory tract. Licorice root is commonly used in herbal teas, tinctures, and lozenges for respiratory congestion and cough relief.

2. **Eucalyptus (Eucalyptus globulus):** Eucalyptus is renowned for its decongestant, antiseptic, and expectorant properties, making it an effective remedy for respiratory congestion and sinusitis. The essential oil of eucalyptus contains cineole, a compound that helps break up mucus and improve airflow in the respiratory tract. Eucalyptus leaf tea, steam inhalation, and chest rubs are popular methods for harnessing its mucus-fighting benefits.

3. **Ginger (Zingiber officinale):** Ginger is prized for its warming, anti-inflammatory, and digestive properties, making it a versatile ingredient in mucus-fighting remedies. It helps alleviate respiratory congestion, soothe sore throats, and support digestion. Ginger can be consumed fresh, as a tea, or in powdered form in capsules or culinary dishes to promote mucus reduction and detoxification.

4. **Turmeric (Curcuma longa):** Turmeric is revered for its potent anti-inflammatory, antioxidant, and immune-modulating properties, making it a valuable addition to mucus-fighting remedies. Curcumin, the active compound in turmeric, helps reduce inflammation in the respiratory tract, support liver detoxification, and alleviate mucus-related symptoms. Turmeric can be consumed fresh, as a spice, or in supplement form to promote respiratory health and mucus clearance.

5. **Peppermint (Mentha piperita):** Peppermint is valued for its cooling, soothing, and decongestant properties, making it an excellent remedy for respiratory congestion and digestive discomfort. Menthol, the primary active compound in peppermint, helps relax bronchial muscles, clear nasal passages, and soothe sore throats. Peppermint tea, steam inhalation, and chest rubs are popular methods for utilizing its mucus-fighting benefits.

Preparing Mucus-Fighting Remedies

Once you have selected your key ingredients for mucus-fighting remedies, it's essential to prepare them in a manner that maximizes their therapeutic potential. Consider the following methods for preparing and using mucus-fighting herbs:

1. **Herbal Teas:** Steep dried or fresh herbs in hot water to create herbal teas that can be sipped throughout the day. Use approximately 1-2 teaspoons of dried herbs or 1-2 tablespoons of fresh herbs per cup of hot water. Allow the herbs to steep for 5-10 minutes, then strain and enjoy the tea warm. Add honey or lemon for flavor and additional respiratory support.

2. **Tinctures:** Tinctures are concentrated herbal extracts made by macerating herbs in alcohol or glycerin to extract their medicinal compounds. Follow dosage recommendations provided by the manufacturer or a qualified herbalist when

using tinctures. Add tinctures to water, juice, or herbal tea for easy consumption and respiratory support.

3. **Steam Inhalation:** Add a few drops of essential oils or dried herbs to a bowl of hot water and inhale the steam to relieve respiratory congestion and promote mucus clearance. Cover your head with a towel and lean over the bowl, keeping your eyes closed to avoid irritation. Breathe deeply for 5-10 minutes, then pat your face dry and rest.

4. **Chest Rubs:** Create homemade chest rubs using infused oils or essential oils of mucus-fighting herbs such as eucalyptus, ginger, and peppermint. Mix the essential oils with a carrier oil such as coconut oil or olive oil, then massage the chest, back, and throat to relieve congestion and soothe respiratory discomfort.

5. **Herbal Baths:** Add dried or fresh herbs to a warm bath to create a soothing herbal infusion that promotes relaxation and respiratory health. Use a muslin bag or cheesecloth to contain the herbs and prevent them from clogging the drain. Soak in the herbal bath for 15-30 minutes, allowing the aromatic steam to penetrate your respiratory system and promote mucus clearance.

Conclusion

In conclusion, selecting and preparing mucus-fighting remedies using key herbal ingredients is a valuable strategy for supporting respiratory health, alleviating congestion, and promoting overall well-being. By harnessing the therapeutic properties of herbs such as licorice root, eucalyptus, ginger, turmeric, and peppermint, individuals can optimize their body's natural detoxification processes and enhance mucus clearance. Experiment with different preparation methods and delivery mechanisms to find what works best for you and your individual needs. As always, consult with a qualified healthcare practitioner or herbalist before starting any herbal regimen, especially if you have underlying health conditions or are taking medications.

CHAPTER EIGHT

Supporting the Body's Natural Healing Processes: Enhancing Immune Function and Digestive Health

Optimal health is intricately linked to the body's ability to support its natural healing processes, which are influenced by various factors including immune function and digestive health. By prioritizing strategies that enhance immune function and support digestive health, individuals can strengthen their body's defenses, promote detoxification, and optimize overall well-being. In this guide, we explore practical ways to support the body's natural healing processes through immune-boosting practices and digestive health strategies.

Enhancing Immune Function

1. **Nutrient-Rich Diet:** Consuming a balanced diet rich in vitamins, minerals, antioxidants, and phytonutrients is essential for supporting immune function. Include a variety of fruits, vegetables, whole grains, lean proteins, and healthy fats in your meals to provide essential nutrients that support immune health.

2. **Immune-Boosting Foods:** Incorporate immune-boosting foods into your diet, such as citrus fruits, berries, leafy greens, garlic, ginger, turmeric, and fermented foods like

yogurt, kefir, sauerkraut, and kimchi. These foods provide vitamins, minerals, and beneficial bacteria that support immune function and promote overall health.

3. **Hydration:** Stay hydrated by drinking plenty of water throughout the day. Hydration is essential for optimal immune function, as it helps flush toxins from the body, supports lymphatic circulation, and maintains mucosal integrity in the respiratory and digestive tracts.

4. **Regular Exercise:** Engage in regular physical activity to support immune function and overall health. Exercise helps boost circulation, reduce inflammation, and promote the production of endorphins, which support immune function and enhance mood.

5. **Stress Management:** Practice stress-reducing techniques such as meditation, deep breathing exercises, yoga, tai chi, and mindfulness to support immune function and promote relaxation. Chronic stress can weaken the immune system and increase susceptibility to illness, so it's essential to prioritize stress management techniques.

6. **Adequate Sleep:** Prioritize quality sleep to support immune function and overall health. Aim for 7-9 hours of sleep per night, as inadequate sleep can impair immune function and increase the risk of illness. Create a relaxing bedtime routine,

limit screen time before bed, and create a comfortable sleep environment to promote restorative sleep.

Supporting Digestive Health

1. **Fiber-Rich Diet:** Consume a diet rich in fiber from fruits, vegetables, whole grains, legumes, nuts, and seeds to support digestive health. Fiber promotes regular bowel movements, prevents constipation, and supports the growth of beneficial gut bacteria.

2. **Probiotic Foods:** Incorporate probiotic-rich foods such as yogurt, kefir, sauerkraut, kimchi, miso, and kombucha into your diet to support gut health and immune function. Probiotics help replenish beneficial gut bacteria, improve digestion, and enhance immune function.

3. **Prebiotic Foods:** Include prebiotic-rich foods such as onions, garlic, leeks, asparagus, bananas, and oats in your diet to support the growth of beneficial gut bacteria. Prebiotics provide fuel for probiotics and help promote a healthy balance of gut flora.

4. **Hydration:** Drink plenty of water throughout the day to support digestion and maintain bowel regularity. Adequate hydration helps soften stools, prevent constipation, and support the movement of waste through the digestive tract.

5. **Limiting Trigger Foods:** Identify and limit foods that may trigger digestive symptoms such as bloating, gas, indigestion, or heartburn. Common trigger foods include spicy foods, greasy foods, caffeine, alcohol, and foods high in refined sugars or artificial additives.

6. **Chewing Thoroughly:** Practice mindful eating and chew your food thoroughly to support digestion and nutrient absorption. Chewing breaks down food into smaller particles, making it easier for digestive enzymes to break down and extract nutrients from food.

Conclusion

In conclusion, supporting the body's natural healing processes through immune-boosting practices and digestive health strategies is essential for promoting overall well-being. By prioritizing nutrient-rich foods, regular exercise, stress management, adequate sleep, and hydration, individuals can strengthen their immune system and support optimal health. Additionally, incorporating fiber-rich foods, probiotics, prebiotics, and mindful eating practices can support digestive health, improve nutrient absorption, and promote bowel regularity. By taking a holistic approach to health and wellness, individuals can empower their body's innate ability to heal and thrive.

CHAPTER NINE

Testimonials of Healing: Inspiring Stories of Individuals Who Have Benefited from Dr. Barbara's Protocol

Dr. Barbara's holistic approach to health and wellness, centered around mucus reduction and detoxification, has touched the lives of many individuals seeking relief from a variety of health challenges. Through her protocol, people have experienced transformative healing journeys, reclaiming vitality, and achieving a renewed sense of well-being. Here are a few inspiring testimonials from individuals who have benefited from Dr. Barbara's protocol:

1. **Sarah's Journey to Respiratory Freedom:** "For years, I struggled with chronic respiratory issues, including frequent congestion, coughing, and sinus infections. Conventional treatments provided temporary relief, but the symptoms always returned. Desperate for a solution, I discovered Dr. Barbara's protocol and decided to give it a try. Within weeks of incorporating herbal remedies, dietary changes, and lifestyle adjustments into my routine, I noticed a significant improvement in my respiratory health. My congestion cleared, my coughing subsided, and I felt like I could breathe freely again. Dr. Barbara's protocol has been a game-changer

for me, giving me the freedom to enjoy life without the burden of constant respiratory discomfort."

2. **Mark's Journey to Digestive Harmony:** "Digestive issues had plagued me for years, leaving me feeling bloated, uncomfortable, and fatigued after meals. I tried numerous diets, medications, and supplements, but nothing seemed to provide lasting relief. That's when I discovered Dr. Barbara's protocol and decided to give it a chance. Through herbal remedies, dietary modifications, and lifestyle changes, I began to notice gradual improvements in my digestive health. Bloating and discomfort became less frequent, and my energy levels soared. Today, I feel more vibrant and alive than ever before, thanks to Dr. Barbara's holistic approach to healing."

3. **Emily's Journey to Vibrant Wellness:** "After years of neglecting my health and indulging in unhealthy habits, I found myself feeling tired, sluggish, and out of balance. I knew I needed to make a change, but I didn't know where to start. That's when I discovered Dr. Barbara's protocol and decided to take control of my health once and for all. Through incorporating mucus-reducing herbs, nourishing foods, and self-care practices into my daily routine, I began to experience a profound transformation. My energy levels increased, my mood improved, and I felt more connected to

my body than ever before. Dr. Barbara's protocol has empowered me to reclaim my health and embrace a vibrant, fulfilling life."

4. **Michael's Journey to Overall Wellness:** "As a busy professional juggling work, family, and personal commitments, I often neglected my health and well-being. Stress, poor dietary choices, and lack of exercise had taken a toll on my body, leaving me feeling depleted and unbalanced. Seeking a holistic solution, I turned to Dr. Barbara's protocol for guidance. Through incorporating herbal remedies, dietary changes, and stress-management techniques into my routine, I began to notice positive changes in my overall health and vitality. I felt more energized, focused, and resilient in the face of life's challenges. Dr. Barbara's protocol has been a beacon of light on my journey to optimal wellness, reminding me to prioritize self-care and embrace a holistic approach to health."

These testimonials reflect the profound impact of Dr. Barbara's protocol on individuals seeking relief from various health concerns. Through a combination of herbal remedies, dietary modifications, lifestyle adjustments, and self-care practices, people have experienced transformative healing journeys, reclaiming vitality, and achieving a renewed sense of well-being.

Dr. Barbara's holistic approach to health and wellness offers hope, inspiration, and empowerment to those on the path to optimal wellness.

CHAPTER TEN

Beyond the Cleanse: Sustaining Health and Wellness Through Long-Term Dietary and Lifestyle Changes

Embarking on a cleanse or detoxification program can provide a powerful reset for the body, but sustaining health and wellness requires long-term dietary and lifestyle changes. Beyond the initial cleanse, adopting sustainable habits is essential for supporting the body's natural detoxification processes, promoting overall well-being, and maintaining vibrant health. In this guide, we explore practical strategies for sustaining health and wellness through long-term dietary and lifestyle changes.

1. Embrace a Whole Foods Diet

Transitioning to a whole foods diet rich in fruits, vegetables, whole grains, lean proteins, and healthy fats is foundational for sustaining health and wellness. Whole foods are nutrient-dense, providing essential vitamins, minerals, antioxidants, and fiber that support detoxification, promote cellular health, and reduce inflammation. Aim to fill your plate with a colorful variety of plant-based foods and minimize consumption of processed foods, refined sugars, and artificial additives.

2. Prioritize Hydration

Staying hydrated is crucial for supporting detoxification, promoting digestion, and maintaining overall health. Aim to drink plenty of water throughout the day, and consider incorporating hydrating foods such as watermelon, cucumber, and citrus fruits into your diet. Herbal teas, coconut water, and freshly pressed juices are also excellent options for staying hydrated and supporting cellular function.

3. Cultivate Gut Health

A healthy gut microbiome is essential for proper digestion, nutrient absorption, and immune function. To support gut health, incorporate probiotic-rich foods such as yogurt, kefir, sauerkraut, and kimchi into your diet. Additionally, consume prebiotic-rich foods such as onions, garlic, asparagus, and bananas to nourish beneficial gut bacteria. Avoiding processed foods, artificial sweeteners, and excessive use of antibiotics can also help maintain a healthy balance of gut flora.

4. Practice Mindful Eating

Mindful eating involves paying attention to your body's hunger and fullness cues, as well as the sensory experience of eating. Slow down and savor each bite, chew your food thoroughly, and eat in a relaxed environment free from distractions. By practicing mindful eating, you can improve digestion, prevent overeating, and cultivate a deeper connection to your body's nutritional needs.

5. Incorporate Regular Physical Activity

Regular physical activity is essential for maintaining cardiovascular health, supporting detoxification, and promoting overall well-being. Find activities that you enjoy and make them a regular part of your routine, whether it's walking, jogging, cycling, yoga, or dancing. Aim for at least 30 minutes of moderate-intensity exercise most days of the week, and incorporate strength training exercises to build muscle mass and support metabolic function.

6. Manage Stress

Chronic stress can have a detrimental effect on health, contributing to inflammation, hormonal imbalances, and digestive issues. Incorporate stress-reducing practices such as meditation, deep breathing exercises, yoga, tai chi, or spending time in nature into your daily routine. Prioritize self-care activities that promote relaxation, rejuvenation, and emotional well-being.

7. Get Adequate Sleep

Quality sleep is essential for cellular repair, hormone regulation, and cognitive function. Aim for 7-9 hours of uninterrupted sleep each night, and create a relaxing bedtime routine to signal to your body that it's time to wind down. Avoid caffeine, electronics, and stimulating activities before bed, and create a comfortable sleep environment that promotes restorative sleep.

8. Practice Gratitude and Positivity

Cultivating a positive mindset and practicing gratitude can have a profound impact on overall health and well-being. Focus on the present moment, find joy in simple pleasures, and express gratitude for the blessings in your life. Surround yourself with supportive relationships, engage in activities that bring you fulfillment, and cultivate a sense of purpose and meaning.

Conclusion

Sustaining health and wellness requires long-term commitment to nourishing the body, mind, and spirit through dietary and lifestyle practices. By embracing a whole foods diet, prioritizing hydration, cultivating gut health, practicing mindful eating, incorporating regular physical activity, managing stress, getting adequate sleep, and fostering positivity, individuals can support their body's natural detoxification processes, promote overall well-being, and thrive in all aspects of life. Remember that sustainable health and wellness are a journey, not a destination, and each positive choice you make contributes to your overall vitality and longevity.

BONUS: SOME ESSENTIAL HERBAL REMEDIES TO KNOW

Bio Ferro Tonic:

Definition: Bio Ferro Tonic is a dietary supplement primarily composed of herbs and minerals. It's often marketed as a natural way to support overall health, particularly by promoting blood health and circulation.

Ingredients: Typical ingredients in Bio Ferro Tonic may include a blend of herbs such as burdock root, yellow dock root, sarsaparilla root, and cascara sagrada bark, along with minerals like iron and potassium phosphate.

How to Prepare: Bio Ferro Tonic usually comes in liquid form and is typically taken orally. It's important to follow the instructions on the product label for dosage and administration.

Dosage: The dosage can vary depending on the specific product and individual needs. It's crucial to consult with a healthcare professional or follow the recommended dosage on the product label to avoid potential side effects.

How to Use: Bio Ferro Tonic is often taken by adding the recommended dosage to water or juice and consuming it orally. It's important to shake the bottle well before use and store it according to the manufacturer's instructions.

Side Effects: While Bio Ferro Tonic is generally considered safe when used as directed, some individuals may experience side effects such as digestive discomfort, allergic reactions, or interactions with medications. It's essential to consult with a healthcare provider before starting any new supplement regimen, especially if you have underlying health conditions or are taking medications.

Blue Vervain:

Definition: Blue vervain, also known as Verbena hastata, is a perennial herb native to North America. It has been used in traditional medicine for centuries to treat various ailments, including anxiety, insomnia, and digestive issues.

Ingredients: Blue vervain contains several active compounds, including aucubin, verbenalin, and volatile oils. These compounds are believed to contribute to the herb's medicinal properties.

How to Prepare: Blue vervain is typically consumed as a tea or tincture. To make tea, dried blue vervain leaves and flowers are steeped in hot water for several minutes before being strained and consumed. Tinctures are prepared by steeping the herb in alcohol or vinegar to extract its active compounds.

Dosage: The appropriate dosage of blue vervain can vary depending on factors such as age, health status, and the specific preparation being used. It's important to follow the recommended dosage on the product label or consult with a qualified herbalist or healthcare professional for personalized guidance.

How to Use: Blue vervain tea or tincture is typically taken orally. It can be consumed on its own or mixed with honey or other herbal teas for added flavor.

Side Effects: While blue vervain is generally considered safe for most people when used in moderation, excessive intake may cause digestive upset or allergic reactions in some individuals. Pregnant or breastfeeding women should avoid blue vervain due to its potential to stimulate uterine contractions. As with any herbal remedy, it's important to consult with a healthcare provider before using blue vervain, especially if you have underlying health conditions or are taking medications.

Bromide Plus Powder:

Definition: Bromide Plus Powder is a dietary supplement formulated to support thyroid health and promote overall well-being. It typically contains a blend of herbs and minerals that are believed to have beneficial effects on thyroid function.

Ingredients: Bromide Plus Powder often contains a combination of herbs such as bladderwrack, sea moss, and burdock root, along with minerals like iodine and potassium phosphate. These ingredients are thought to support thyroid function and maintain optimal iodine levels in the body.

How to Prepare: Bromide Plus Powder is usually mixed with water or juice to create a drinkable solution. It's important to follow the instructions on the product label for dosage and preparation.

Dosage: The dosage of Bromide Plus Powder can vary depending on the specific product and individual needs. It's crucial to consult with a healthcare professional or follow the recommended dosage on the product label to avoid potential side effects.

How to Use: Bromide Plus Powder is typically taken orally by mixing the recommended dosage with water or juice. It's important to shake or stir the mixture well before consuming it to ensure even distribution of the ingredients.

Side Effects: While Bromide Plus Powder is generally considered safe when used as directed, some individuals may experience side effects such as digestive discomfort or allergic reactions to certain ingredients. It's essential to consult with a healthcare provider before starting any new supplement regimen, especially if you have underlying health conditions or are taking medications.

Bugleweed:

Definition: Bugleweed, also known as Lycopusvirginicus, is a perennial herb native to North America and Europe. It has been used in traditional medicine to treat various conditions, including hyperthyroidism, anxiety, and insomnia.

Ingredients: Bugleweed contains several active compounds, including lithospermic acid, phenolic acids, and flavonoids. These compounds are believed to contribute to the herb's medicinal properties, particularly its ability to regulate thyroid function.

How to Prepare: Bugleweed is commonly consumed as a tea or tincture. To make tea, dried bugleweed leaves and flowers are steeped in hot water for several minutes before being strained and consumed. Tinctures are prepared by steeping the herb in alcohol or vinegar to extract its active compounds.

Dosage: The appropriate dosage of bugleweed can vary depending on factors such as age, health status, and the specific preparation being used. It's important to follow the recommended dosage on the product label or consult with a qualified herbalist or healthcare professional for personalized guidance.

How to Use: Bugleweed tea or tincture is typically taken orally. It can be consumed on its own or mixed with honey or other herbal teas for added flavor.

Side Effects: While bugleweed is generally considered safe for most people when used in moderation, excessive intake may cause digestive upset or allergic reactions in some individuals.

Pregnant or breastfeeding women should avoid bugleweed due to its potential to stimulate uterine contractions. As with any herbal remedy, it's important to consult with a healthcare provider before using bugleweed, especially if you have underlying health conditions or are taking medications.

Burdock:

Definition: Burdock, scientifically known as Arctium lappa, is a biennial plant native to Europe and Asia but now found worldwide. It's part of the Asteraceae family and has been used for centuries in traditional medicine and culinary practices.

Ingredients: Burdock contains various nutrients, including carbohydrates, fiber, vitamins (such as vitamin B6, folate, and vitamin C), and minerals (including potassium, magnesium, and manganese). It also contains active compounds such as polyphenols and volatile oils.

How to Prepare: Burdock can be prepared and consumed in various ways. The roots, leaves, and seeds are all utilized for different purposes. The root is commonly used in cooking, herbal teas, tinctures, and supplements, while the leaves and seeds are sometimes used in herbal preparations.

Dosage: The appropriate dosage of burdock root can vary depending on the specific form and intended use. For culinary purposes, there are no strict dosage guidelines, but for supplements or herbal remedies, it's essential to follow the recommended dosage on the product label or consult with a healthcare professional.

How to Use: Burdock root can be used in cooking by peeling, slicing, and adding it to soups, stews, stir-fries, or salads. It can also be brewed into a tea or used to make tinctures or extracts for medicinal purposes. Some people may also take burdock root supplements in capsule or powder form.

Side Effects: While burdock is generally considered safe for most people when consumed in moderate amounts, some individuals may experience allergic reactions or digestive upset. Additionally, burdock may interact with certain medications or have adverse effects in individuals with certain health conditions, such as diabetes or allergies to plants in the Asteraceae family. It's important to consult with a healthcare provider before using burdock, especially if you have underlying health conditions or are taking medications.

Cascara Sagrada:

Definition: Cascara Sagrada, scientifically known as Rhamnus purshiana, is a species of buckthorn native to western North America. It has been used traditionally as a laxative and to promote bowel regularity.

Ingredients: The primary active ingredients in cascara sagrada are anthraquinone glycosides, particularly cascarosides A and B. These compounds stimulate peristalsis in the colon, leading to increased bowel movements.

How to Prepare: Cascara sagrada is typically prepared as an herbal tea, tincture, or capsule. To make tea, dried cascara sagrada bark is steeped in hot water for several minutes before being strained and consumed. Tinctures are prepared by steeping the bark in alcohol to extract its active compounds.

Dosage: The appropriate dosage of cascara sagrada can vary depending on the specific preparation and intended use. It's important to follow the recommended dosage on the product label or consult with a healthcare professional for personalized guidance.

How to Use: Cascara sagrada tea or tincture is typically taken orally. It's important to start with a low dose and gradually increase if needed to avoid potential side effects such as cramping or diarrhea.

Side Effects: Cascara sagrada is considered safe for short-term use when used as directed. However, long-term or excessive use may lead to dependence, electrolyte imbalance, or dehydration. It may also interact with certain medications or have adverse effects in individuals with certain health conditions. It's important to use cascara sagrada under the guidance of a healthcare professional and to discontinue use if any adverse effects occur.

Cell Food:

Definition: Cell Food is a dietary supplement marketed as a highly oxygenating and alkalizing formula. It's claimed to support overall health and vitality by providing essential nutrients and oxygen to the cells.

Ingredients: The exact ingredients of Cell Food can vary depending on the brand, but it typically contains a proprietary blend of minerals, enzymes, electrolytes, and trace elements. Some common ingredients may include purified water, dissolved oxygen, seawater extract, and plant-based enzymes.

How to Prepare: Cell Food is usually available in liquid form and is typically taken orally. It can be consumed directly or diluted in water or juice before consumption.

Dosage: The dosage of Cell Food can vary depending on the specific product and individual needs. It's important to follow the recommended dosage on the product label or consult with a healthcare professional for personalized guidance.

How to Use: Cell Food is typically taken orally, either directly or mixed into water or juice. It's important to shake the bottle well before use and to store it according to the manufacturer's instructions.

Side Effects: Cell Food is generally considered safe for most people when used as directed. However, some individuals may experience mild digestive upset or allergic reactions to certain ingredients. It's essential to consult with a healthcare provider before starting any new supplement regimen, especially if you have underlying health conditions or are taking medications.

Chaparral:

Definition: Chaparral, scientifically known as Larrea tridentata, is a shrub native to the southwestern United States and northern Mexico. It has been used for centuries by Native American tribes for its medicinal properties and is commonly used in herbal medicine today.

Ingredients: Chaparral contains several bioactive compounds, including nordihydroguaiaretic acid (NDGA), flavonoids, lignans, and volatile oils. NDGA is believed to be the primary active compound responsible for many of chaparral's therapeutic effects.

How to Prepare: Chaparral can be prepared and consumed in various forms, including teas, tinctures, capsules, and topical preparations. To make tea, dried chaparral leaves are steeped in hot water for several minutes before being strained and consumed. Tinctures are prepared by steeping the herb in alcohol or vinegar to extract its active compounds.

Dosage: The appropriate dosage of chaparral can vary depending on the specific form and intended use. It's important to follow the recommended dosage on the product label or consult with a healthcare professional for personalized guidance.

How to Use: Chaparral tea or tincture is typically taken orally. It can also be applied topically to the skin for certain conditions. It's important to use chaparral products as directed and to discontinue use if any adverse effects occur.

Side Effects: Chaparral is generally considered safe for most people when used in moderate amounts. However, excessive intake or prolonged use may lead to liver toxicity or other adverse effects. It may also interact with certain medications or have adverse effects in individuals with certain health conditions. It's important to use chaparral under the guidance of a healthcare professional and to discontinue use if any adverse effects occur.

Cocolmeca:

Definition: Cocolmeca, also known as Smilax ornata or sarsaparilla, is a flowering vine native to Mexico and Central America. It has been used traditionally in Mexican and Central American folk medicine for its purported medicinal properties.

Ingredients: Cocolmeca contains various bioactive compounds, including saponins, flavonoids, and plant sterols. These compounds are believed to contribute to the herb's medicinal properties, including its potential as a diuretic, blood purifier, and anti-inflammatory agent.

How to Prepare: Cocolmeca is commonly prepared and consumed as an herbal tea or decoction. To make tea, dried cocolmeca roots or leaves are steeped in hot water for several minutes before being strained and consumed. Decoctions involve boiling the roots or leaves in water to extract their active compounds.

Dosage: The appropriate dosage of cocolmeca can vary depending on factors such as age, health status, and the specific preparation being used. It's important to follow the recommended dosage on the product label or consult with a qualified herbalist or healthcare professional for personalized guidance.

How to Use: Cocolmeca tea or decoction is typically taken orally. It can also be used topically for certain skin conditions. It's important to use cocolmeca products as directed and to discontinue use if any adverse effects occur.

Side Effects: Cocolmeca is generally considered safe for most people when used in moderate amounts. However, excessive intake may lead to digestive upset or other adverse effects. It may also interact with certain medications or have adverse effects in individuals with certain health conditions. It's important to use cocolmeca under the guidance of a healthcare professional and to discontinue use if any adverse effects occur.

Contribo:

Definition: Contribo, also known as Aristolochiatrilobata, is a vine native to the Caribbean and Central America. It has been used traditionally in folk medicine for various purposes, including as a remedy for digestive issues, inflammation, and pain relief.

Ingredients: Contribo contains several bioactive compounds, including aristolochic acids, flavonoids, and alkaloids. These compounds are believed to contribute to the herb's medicinal properties, including its potential as an anti-inflammatory and analgesic agent.

How to Prepare: Contribo is typically prepared and consumed as an herbal tea or decoction. To make tea, dried contribo leaves or stems are steeped in hot water for several minutes before being strained and consumed. Decoctions involve boiling the leaves or stems in water to extract their active compounds.

Dosage: The appropriate dosage of contribo can vary depending on factors such as age, health status, and the specific preparation being used. It's important to follow the recommended dosage on the product label or consult with a qualified herbalist or healthcare professional for personalized guidance.

How to Use: Contribo tea or decoction is typically taken orally. It's important to use contribo products as directed and to discontinue use if any adverse effects occur.

Side Effects: Contribo contains aristolochic acids, which have been associated with serious adverse effects, including kidney damage and cancer. Due to these safety concerns, the use of contribo is highly discouraged, and it's important to avoid products containing aristolochic acids. Individuals should seek alternative remedies for their health needs.

Dandelion Root:

Definition: Dandelion, scientifically known as Taraxacum officinale, is a common flowering plant found worldwide. While often considered a pesky weed, dandelion has a long history of use in traditional medicine for its various health benefits.

Ingredients: Dandelion root contains several bioactive compounds, including sesquiterpene lactones, triterpenes, flavonoids, and polysaccharides. These compounds are believed to contribute to the herb's medicinal properties, including its potential as a diuretic, digestive aid, and liver tonic.

How to Prepare: Dandelion root can be prepared and consumed in various forms, including teas, tinctures, capsules, and extracts. To make tea, dried dandelion root is steeped in hot water for several minutes before being strained and consumed. Tinctures are prepared by steeping the root in alcohol or vinegar to extract its active compounds.

Dosage: The appropriate dosage of dandelion root can vary depending on factors such as age, health status, and the specific preparation being used. It's important to follow the recommended dosage on the product label or consult with a qualified herbalist or healthcare professional for personalized guidance.

How to Use: Dandelion root tea, tincture, or capsules are typically taken orally. It's important to use dandelion root products as directed and to discontinue use if any adverse effects occur.

Side Effects: Dandelion root is generally considered safe for most people when used in moderate amounts. However, some individuals may experience allergic reactions or digestive upset. It may also interact with certain medications or have adverse effects in individuals with certain health conditions. It's important to use dandelion root under the guidance of a healthcare professional and to discontinue use if any adverse effects occur.

Green Food Plus:

Definition: Green Food Plus is a dietary supplement formulated to provide a concentrated source of nutrients derived from various green plants. It's designed to support overall health and well-being by delivering essential vitamins, minerals, antioxidants, and phytonutrients.

Ingredients: Green Food Plus typically contains a blend of powdered green vegetables, grasses, algae, and other plant-based ingredients. Common ingredients may include wheatgrass, barley grass, spirulina, chlorella, alfalfa, kale, spinach, and broccoli, among others.

How to Prepare: Green Food Plus is usually available in powder form and can be mixed with water, juice, or smoothies. It's important to follow the recommended dosage on the product label and to consume it as part of a balanced diet.

Dosage: The appropriate dosage of Green Food Plus can vary depending on the specific product and individual needs. It's important to follow the recommended dosage on the product label or consult with a healthcare professional for personalized guidance.

How to Use: Green Food Plus powder is typically mixed with water, juice, or smoothies and consumed orally. It's often taken once or twice daily, preferably with meals, to maximize nutrient absorption.

Side Effects: Green Food Plus is generally considered safe for most people when used as directed. However, some individuals may experience digestive upset or allergic reactions to certain ingredients. It's important to consult with a healthcare provider before starting any new supplement regimen, especially if you have underlying health conditions or are taking medications.

Irish Moss:

Definition: Irish Moss, scientifically known as Chondrus crispus, is a species of red algae or seaweed native to the Atlantic coastlines of Europe and North America. It has been used for centuries in traditional Irish and Scottish cuisine, as well as in herbal medicine.

Ingredients: Irish Moss is rich in various nutrients, including iodine, sulfur compounds, vitamins (such as vitamin A, vitamin K, and vitamin B12), minerals (including calcium, magnesium, potassium, and sodium), and polysaccharides (such as carrageenan). These nutrients are believed to contribute to the herb's potential health benefits.

How to Prepare: Irish Moss is typically prepared by soaking it in water to rehydrate and soften it before use. It can be added to soups, stews, smoothies, desserts, and other dishes as a thickening agent or nutritional supplement.

Dosage: The appropriate dosage of Irish Moss can vary depending on factors such as age, health status, and the specific preparation being used. It's important to follow recipes or guidelines for culinary use and to consult with a healthcare professional for guidance on using Irish Moss as a dietary supplement.

How to Use: Irish Moss can be used in culinary applications to add thickness and nutritional value to dishes. It can also be consumed as a dietary supplement in the form of capsules, powders, or extracts.

Side Effects: Irish Moss is generally considered safe for most people when consumed in moderate amounts as part of a balanced diet. However, some individuals may be allergic to seaweed or carrageenan, a compound found in Irish Moss that is used as a food additive. It's important to discontinue use if any adverse effects occur and to consult with a healthcare professional if you have any concerns.

Irish Sea Moss:

Definition: Irish Sea Moss is a term often used interchangeably with Irish Moss, referring to the same species of red algae, Chondrus crispus. It's harvested from the rocky shores of the Atlantic coastlines of Europe and North America.

Ingredients: Irish Sea Moss shares the same nutritional profile as Irish Moss, containing iodine, vitamins, minerals, and polysaccharides. It's valued for its potential health benefits, including supporting thyroid function, boosting immune health, and promoting digestion.

How to Prepare: Irish Sea Moss is prepared in the same way as Irish Moss, by soaking it in water to rehydrate and soften it before use. It can be used in culinary applications or consumed as a dietary supplement.

Dosage: The dosage of Irish Sea Moss depends on the form and intended use. As a dietary supplement, it's important to follow the recommended dosage on the product label or consult with a healthcare professional for personalized guidance.

How to Use: Irish Sea Moss can be used in various culinary applications, including soups, smoothies, desserts, and sauces. It can also be consumed as a dietary supplement in the form of capsules, powders, or extracts.

Side Effects: Similar to Irish Moss, Irish Sea Moss is generally considered safe for most people when consumed in moderate amounts. However, individuals with seaweed allergies or sensitivities to carrageenan should exercise caution. It's important to discontinue use if any adverse effects occur and to consult with a healthcare professional if you have any concerns.

Lymphalin:

Definition: Lymphalin is a herbal supplement formulated to support lymphatic system health. The lymphatic system plays a crucial role in immune function and waste removal in the body, and Lymphalin is designed to promote its proper function.

Ingredients: Lymphalin typically contains a blend of herbs and botanical extracts known for their traditional use in supporting lymphatic system health. Common ingredients may include cleavers, red clover, echinacea, burdock root, and calendula, among others.

How to Prepare: Lymphalin is usually available in capsule or liquid form. Capsules are taken orally with water, while liquid forms may be mixed with water or juice before consumption. It's important to follow the recommended dosage on the product label.

Dosage: The appropriate dosage of Lymphalin can vary depending on the specific product and individual needs. It's important to follow the recommended dosage on the product label or consult with a healthcare professional for personalized guidance.

How to Use: Lymphalin capsules are typically taken orally with water, while liquid forms may be mixed with water or juice before consumption. It's often recommended to take Lymphalin on an empty stomach for optimal absorption.

Side Effects: Lymphalin is generally considered safe for most people when used as directed. However, some individuals may experience mild side effects such as gastrointestinal discomfort or allergic reactions to certain ingredients. It's important to consult with a healthcare provider before starting any new supplement regimen, especially if you have underlying health conditions or are taking medications.

Manjakani:

Definition: Manjakani, also known as Quercus infectoria or oak gall, is a natural substance derived from the oak tree. It has been used for centuries in traditional medicine for its potential health benefits, particularly for women's health and vaginal tightening.

Ingredients: Manjakani contains various bioactive compounds, including tannins, flavonoids, and gallic acid. These compounds are believed to contribute to the herb's medicinal properties, including its potential as an astringent and antiseptic agent.

How to Prepare: Manjakani is typically available in powder, capsule, or liquid extract form. It can be taken orally or used topically depending on the intended use. For vaginal tightening, manjakani may be applied topically as a gel or inserted into the vagina in capsule form.

Dosage: The appropriate dosage of manjakani can vary depending on factors such as age, health status, and the specific preparation being used. It's important to follow the recommended dosage on the product label or consult with a qualified herbalist or healthcare professional for personalized guidance.

How to Use: Manjakani can be taken orally or used topically depending on the intended use. It's important to use manjakani products as directed and to discontinue use if any adverse effects occur.

Side Effects: Manjakani is generally considered safe for most people when used in moderate amounts. However, some individuals may experience allergic reactions or skin irritation when used topically. It's important to use manjakani under the guidance of a healthcare professional and to discontinue use if any adverse effects occur.

Red Clover:

Definition: Red clover, scientifically known as Trifolium pratense, is a flowering plant belonging to the legume family. It's native to Europe, Western Asia, and Northwest Africa but has been naturalized in many other regions. Red clover has been used in traditional medicine for various purposes, including its potential to support women's health and menopausal symptoms.

Ingredients: Red clover contains several bioactive compounds, including isoflavones (such as genistein and daidzein), flavonoids, and phytoestrogens. These compounds are believed to contribute to the herb's medicinal properties, including its potential as a hormone-balancing agent and its ability to support cardiovascular health.

How to Prepare: Red clover is typically prepared and consumed as an herbal tea or tincture. To make tea, dried red clover flowers are steeped in hot water for several minutes before being strained and consumed. Tinctures are prepared by steeping the flowers in alcohol or vinegar to extract their active compounds.

Dosage: The appropriate dosage of red clover can vary depending on factors such as age, health status, and the specific preparation being used. It's important to follow the recommended dosage on the product label or consult with a qualified herbalist or healthcare professional for personalized guidance.

How to Use: Red clover tea or tincture is typically taken orally. It's important to use red clover products as directed and to discontinue use if any adverse effects occur.

Side Effects: Red clover is generally considered safe for most people when used in moderate amounts. However, some individuals may experience allergic reactions or digestive upset. It may also interact with certain medications or have adverse effects in individuals with certain health conditions. It's important to use red clover under the guidance of a healthcare professional and to discontinue use if any adverse effects occur.

Guaco:

Definition: Guaco, also known as Mikania cordata or Mikania glomerata, is a medicinal plant native to Central and South America. It has a long history of use in traditional medicine for its potential therapeutic properties.

Ingredients: Guaco contains several bioactive compounds, including coumarins, flavonoids, tannins, and saponins. These compounds are believed to contribute to the herb's medicinal properties, including its potential as an expectorant, anti-inflammatory, and antispasmodic agent.

How to Prepare: Guaco is typically prepared and consumed as an herbal tea or infusion. To make tea, dried guaco leaves are steeped in hot water for several minutes before being strained and consumed.

Dosage: The appropriate dosage of guaco can vary depending on factors such as age, health status, and the specific preparation being used. It's important to follow the recommended dosage on the product label or consult with a qualified herbalist or healthcare professional for personalized guidance.

How to Use: Guaco tea is typically taken orally. It can be consumed on its own or mixed with honey or other herbal teas for added flavor.

Side Effects: Guaco is generally considered safe for most people when used in moderate amounts. However, some individuals may experience allergic reactions or digestive upset. It may also interact with certain medications or have adverse effects in individuals with certain health conditions. It's important to use guaco under the guidance of a healthcare professional and to discontinue use if any adverse effects occur.

Herban Iron:

Definition: Herban Iron is a dietary supplement designed to provide an easily absorbable form of iron to support healthy iron levels in the body. It's particularly beneficial for individuals with iron deficiency or anemia.

Ingredients: Herban Iron typically contains iron in the form of ferrous bisglycinate, which is a highly bioavailable and gentle form of iron that is less likely to cause digestive upset or constipation compared to other forms of iron. It may also contain other ingredients such as vitamin C to enhance iron absorption.

How to Prepare: Herban Iron is usually available in capsule or liquid form. Capsules are taken orally with water, while liquid forms may be mixed with water or juice before consumption. It's important to follow the recommended dosage on the product label.

Dosage: The appropriate dosage of Herban Iron depends on factors such as age, gender, and the severity of iron deficiency. It's important to consult with a healthcare professional to determine the correct dosage for individual needs.

How to Use: Herban Iron capsules are typically taken orally with water, while liquid forms may be mixed with water or juice before consumption. It's important to take Herban Iron as directed and to avoid taking it with dairy products, antacids, or other substances that may interfere with iron absorption.

Side Effects: While Herban Iron is generally considered safe for most people when used as directed, some individuals may experience mild side effects such as gastrointestinal discomfort or constipation. It's important to consult with a healthcare professional before starting any new supplement regimen, especially if you have underlying health conditions or are taking medications.

Hydrangea:

Definition: Hydrangea, scientifically known as Hydrangea arborescens, is a flowering shrub native to North America. It has been used traditionally in herbal medicine for its potential diuretic and anti-inflammatory properties.

Ingredients: Hydrangea contains several bioactive compounds, including saponins, flavonoids, and glycosides. These compounds are believed to contribute to the herb's medicinal properties, including its potential as a diuretic, kidney tonic, and anti-inflammatory agent.

How to Prepare: Hydrangea root is typically prepared and consumed as an herbal tea or tincture. To make tea, dried hydrangea root is steeped in hot water for several minutes before being strained and consumed. Tinctures are prepared by steeping the root in alcohol or vinegar to extract its active compounds.

Dosage: The appropriate dosage of hydrangea can vary depending on factors such as age, health status, and the specific preparation being used. It's important to follow the recommended dosage on the product label or consult with a qualified herbalist or healthcare professional for personalized guidance.

How to Use: Hydrangea tea or tincture is typically taken orally. It's important to use hydrangea products as directed and to discontinue use if any adverse effects occur.

Side Effects: Hydrangea is generally considered safe for most people when used in moderate amounts. However, some individuals may experience digestive upset or allergic reactions. It may also interact with certain medications or have adverse effects in individuals with certain health conditions. It's important to use hydrangea under the guidance of a healthcare professional and to discontinue use if any adverse effects occur.

Bladderwrack:

Definition: Bladderwrack is a type of seaweed or marine algae commonly used in traditional medicine and as a dietary supplement. It's known for its potential health benefits, particularly related to thyroid health and weight management.

Ingredients: Bladderwrack contains various nutrients, including iodine, vitamins, minerals, and antioxidants. The primary active components are iodine and fucoidan, a type of carbohydrate found in brown seaweeds.

How to Prepare: Bladderwrack supplements are available in various forms, including capsules, powders, and liquid extracts. They can be taken orally with water or added to smoothies and other beverages.

Dosage: The appropriate dosage of bladderwrack can vary based on factors such as age, health status, and the specific product being used. It's essential to follow the recommended dosage on the product label or consult with a healthcare professional for personalized guidance.

How to Use: Bladderwrack supplements are typically taken orally, either with water or mixed into food or beverages. It's important to follow the instructions on the product label and avoid exceeding the recommended dosage.

Side Effects: While bladderwrack is generally considered safe for most people when used in moderation, excessive intake of iodine from bladderwrack supplements can cause thyroid dysfunction and other adverse effects. Individuals with thyroid disorders, iodine sensitivity, or certain medical conditions should exercise caution and consult with a healthcare provider before using bladderwrack supplements. Common side effects may include digestive upset, allergic reactions, or interactions with medications.

Blood Purifier:

Definition: Blood purifiers are herbal remedies or dietary supplements believed to cleanse or detoxify the blood, often promoting overall health and well-being. They are thought to support the body's natural detoxification processes and improve blood circulation.

Ingredients: Blood purifiers may contain a variety of herbs and botanical extracts known for their purported cleansing and detoxifying properties. Common ingredients include burdock root, red clover, dandelion root, and yellow dock root, among others.

How to Prepare: Blood purifiers are typically available in various forms, including capsules, tablets, powders, and liquid extracts. They are usually taken orally with water or juice, following the recommended dosage on the product label.

Dosage: The dosage of blood purifiers can vary depending on the specific product and individual needs. It's important to adhere to the recommended dosage on the product label or consult with a healthcare professional for personalized guidance.

How to Use: Blood purifiers are typically taken orally, either with water or mixed into beverages. They are often used as part of a detoxification regimen or to support overall health and vitality.

Side Effects: While blood purifiers are generally considered safe for most people when used as directed, some individuals may experience side effects such as digestive discomfort, allergic reactions, or interactions with medications. It's important to consult with a healthcare provider before starting any new supplement regimen, especially if you have underlying health conditions or are taking medications.

THE END